REVITALIZE AND TONE:

30 DAYS CHAIR PILATES FOR WOMEN IN THEIR 40s AND BEYOND"

By
Chris Elliot

Preface:

A Journey to Revitalize and Tone

In a bustling city filled with women in their 40s and beyond, a sense of vitality and rejuvenation was calling out to them. They yearned to embrace their bodies, strengthen their cores, and embark on a journey towards improved fitness and well-being. It was in this vibrant community that the concept of Chair Pilates began to take shape.

Revitalize and Tone: Chair Pilates for Women in Their 40s and Beyond is a book born from the desire to empower and uplift women as they navigate the beautiful and transformative phase of life. It is a tale of discovery, self-care, and the incredible potential that lies within each individual.

Within these pages, you will find a collection of carefully curated exercises, routines, and guidance specifically designed to cater to the unique needs of women in their 40s and beyond. Chair Pilates, with its gentle yet effective approach, becomes the perfect companion on this journey of revitalization.

As the story unfolds, you will delve into the art of mindful movement, exploring the power of a sturdy chair as your support system. Each exercise, each stretch, and each routine serves as a stepping stone towards enhanced strength, flexibility, balance, and improved posture.

But this is not just a book about physical transformation; it is an invitation to embrace self-care and self-discovery. It encourages you to listen to your body, honor its needs, and build a deeper connection with yourself. Through the magic of Chair Pilates, you will learn to rekindle your inner fire, ignite your confidence, and embrace the fullness of life.

In the chapters that follow, you will embark on a remarkable journey of revitalization and toning. From an energizing morning routine that kickstarts your day to a midday recharge and an evening relaxation routine that help you find inner calmness, you will discover the power of these movements to elevate your well-being.

This book is not merely a manual; it is an enchanting tale that unfolds as you turn each page. It is a reminder that age is but a number, and that every woman, regardless of where she is in her life's journey, deserves to thrive, flourish, and feel radiant.

So, dear reader, I invite you to join us on this captivating adventure. Embrace the story that awaits within these chapters, and let Chair Pilates be your guide to revitalization, toning, and a newfound sense of vitality. May this book inspire you to embark on your own transformative journey, as you reclaim your strength, nurture your body, and discover the incredible power that lies within you. Let the tale begin!

Copyright

Table of Contents:

CHAPTER 1. INTRODUCTION TO CHAIR PILATES FOR WOMEN OVER 40 AND BEYOND

Introduction

Welcome to the world of Chair Pilates! This book is specifically designed to introduce women over 40 to the benefits of practicing Pilates on a chair. As we age, maintaining strength, flexibility, and overall well-being becomes increasingly important. Chair Pilates offers a safe and effective exercise method that can help improve posture, increase muscle tone, and enhance overall body awareness.

Chair Pilates takes the principles and exercises of traditional Pilates and adapts them to be performed on a chair, making it accessible for women of all fitness levels. The chair provides stability and support, allowing individuals to focus on proper alignment and controlled movements. This low-impact form of exercise is gentle on the joints while still challenging the muscles.

In this book, we will explore essential equipment and setup for Chair Pilates, as well as foundational exercises that target the core, upper body, and lower body. You will also discover exercises to enhance flexibility and balance, along with chair Pilates routines for daily practice.

Whether you are new to Pilates or have some prior experience, Chair Pilates will provide you with a comprehensive guide to help you improve strength, flexibility, and overall fitness. Get ready to embark on a journey of rejuvenation, empowerment, and well-being. Let's begin!

GETTING STARTED: ESSENTIAL EQUIPMENT AND SETUP

Before diving into Chair Pilates, it's important to ensure you have the necessary equipment and set up your space properly. Here are some essential considerations to get you started:

1. Chair Selection: Choose a sturdy, armless chair with a straight back and a stable base. Avoid chairs with wheels or cushions that may compromise stability during exercises.

2. Clear Space: Clear a designated area in your home where you can comfortably perform your Chair Pilates exercises. Ensure there is ample room around the chair to move freely without any obstructions.

3. Proper Clothing: Wear comfortable clothing that allows for unrestricted movement. Opt for breathable fabrics that stretch with your body and avoid anything too loose or constricting.

4. Footwear: Perform Chair Pilates barefoot or wear grip socks to prevent slipping. Avoid

shoes with thick soles as they may affect your stability and balance.

5. Props and Accessories: Gather any additional props or accessories you may want to incorporate, such as resistance bands, small weights, or a cushion for added comfort.

6. Warm-Up: Prior to starting your Chair Pilates session, consider incorporating a brief warm-up routine to prepare your muscles and joints for exercise. This can include light cardio movements, gentle stretches, or deep breathing exercises.

Remember, safety and comfort are key when setting up your Chair Pilates space. By ensuring you have the right equipment and a suitable environment, you can fully focus on your practice and maximize the benefits of your workouts. Now that you're set up, let's delve into the invigorating world of Chair Pilates!

CHAPTER 2. CHAIR PILATES EXERCISES FOR STRENGTH AND FLEXIBILITY

- Core Strengthening And Stability Exercises

One of the key focuses of Chair Pilates is to strengthen and stabilize the core muscles, which includes the muscles of the abdomen, lower back, and pelvis. A strong core not only enhances your posture and balance but also supports and protects your spine during daily activities. Here are some core strengthening and stability exercises you can perform on a chair:

1. Seated Spinal Twist: Sit tall on the chair with your feet planted firmly on the ground. Place

your right hand on the outside of your left thigh and your left hand on the backrest of the chair. Inhale to lengthen your spine, then exhale as you twist your torso to the left, using your hands to gently deepen the stretch. Hold for a few breaths, then repeat on the other side.

2. Abdominal Scoop: Sit on the edge of the chair, feet hip-width apart and flat on the floor. Place your hands on the sides of the chair, fingers pointing forward. Inhale deeply, then as you exhale, engage your abdominal muscles and slowly round your spine, scooping your belly inwards. Hold this position for a few seconds, then release and repeat.

3. Knee Lifts: Sit on the chair with your hands resting lightly on the sides of the chair seat. Keep your back straight and engage your core. Lift your right knee towards your chest, maintaining a controlled movement. Slowly lower it back down and repeat with the left knee. Continue alternating legs for a set number of repetitions.

4. Pelvic Tilts: Sit on the chair with your feet flat on the floor and hip-width apart. Place your hands on your hips. Inhale deeply, then as you exhale, tilt your pelvis forward, pressing your lower back into the chair. Hold for a few seconds, then inhale and release the tilt, allowing your lower back to arch slightly. Repeat the movement, focusing on engaging your core and maintaining control.

5. Side Plank with Chair Support: Sit on the edge of the chair and place your right hand on the seat, fingers pointing towards the side. Extend your legs to the left, keeping them stacked on top of each other. Lift your hips off the chair, creating a straight line from head to heels. Hold for a few breaths, then lower your hips back down. Repeat on the other side.

Remember to maintain proper form and alignment throughout these exercises. Focus on engaging your core muscles and performing the movements with control and precision. Gradually increase the intensity and duration of the exercises as your core strength improves. Core strengthening and stability exercises on a chair can be a challenging and effective way to build a strong foundation for your overall fitness and well-being.

- *Upper Body And Arm Exercises*

Incorporating upper body and arm exercises into your Chair Pilates routine helps strengthen and tone the muscles in your arms, shoulders, and upper back. These exercises will enhance your posture, improve upper body strength, and promote better functional movement. Here are some upper body and arm exercises you can perform on a chair:

1. Arm Circles: Sit tall on the chair with your feet flat on the floor. Extend your arms straight out to the sides at shoulder height. Begin by making small circles with your arms, gradually increasing the size of the circles. After a few rotations, change the direction of the circles. Focus on engaging your shoulder blades and maintaining good posture throughout the movement.

2. Triceps Dips: Sit on the edge of the chair and place your hands on the seat, fingers pointing forward. Slide your bottom off the chair, keeping your hands shoulder-width apart. Bend your elbows and lower your body towards the floor, then push through your hands to straighten your arms and lift your body back up. Repeat this dip motion, focusing on engaging your triceps.

3. Shoulder Press: Sit tall on the chair with your feet flat on the floor. Hold a pair of small weights (or water bottles) in your hands, with your elbows bent and palms facing forward. Inhale deeply, then as you exhale, extend your arms overhead, fully straightening them without locking your elbows. Inhale to lower your arms back down to the starting position. Repeat for a set number of repetitions.

4. Bicep Curls: Sit tall on the chair with your feet flat on the floor and a weight in each hand, palms facing forward. Keeping your upper arms still, bend your elbows and lift the weights towards your shoulders. Pause for a moment,

then slowly lower the weights back down. Focus on engaging your biceps and maintaining control throughout the movement.

5. Chest Opener: Sit tall on the chair with your feet flat on the floor. Interlace your fingers behind your back, squeezing your shoulder blades together. Inhale deeply, then as you exhale, gently lift your interlaced hands away from your body, opening your chest. Hold for a few breaths, then release and repeat.

These upper body and arm exercises can be tailored to your fitness level by adjusting the weight or intensity. Start with a weight that challenges you without compromising your form, and gradually increase the resistance as you build strength. Remember to maintain proper posture, engage your core, and perform the movements with control. By incorporating these exercises into your Chair Pilates routine, you'll improve your upper body strength, posture, and overall muscular balance.

- Lower Body Sculpting And Toning

Targeting the lower body through Chair Pilates exercises is an excellent way to sculpt and tone your legs, glutes, and hips. These exercises will help strengthen and lengthen your muscles, improve stability, and enhance overall lower body strength and flexibility. Here are some lower body sculpting and toning exercises you can perform on a chair:

1. Chair Squats: Stand in front of the chair with your feet hip-width apart. Extend your arms forward for balance. Inhale as you sit back into a squat, lowering your hips towards the chair while keeping your knees in line with your toes. Exhale and push through your heels to stand back up. Repeat for a set number of repetitions, focusing on engaging your glutes and quadriceps.

2. Leg Extensions: Sit tall on the chair with your feet flat on the floor. Extend one leg straight out in front of you, squeezing your quadriceps (front thigh muscles) as you do so. Hold for a moment, then lower your foot back down.

Repeat on the other leg. To increase the challenge, you can add ankle weights or use a resistance band around your ankles.

3. Inner Thigh Squeezes: Sit on the chair with your knees bent and feet flat on the floor. Place a small pillow or a soft ball between your knees. Inhale deeply, then as you exhale, squeeze the pillow or ball with your inner thighs. Hold the squeeze for a few seconds, then release. Repeat for a set number of repetitions, focusing on engaging your inner thigh muscles.

4. Glute Bridge: Sit on the edge of the chair with your feet planted firmly on the floor and hip-width apart. Place your hands on the sides of the chair for support. Inhale deeply, then as you exhale, press through your heels and lift your hips off the chair, creating a straight line from your knees to your shoulders. Hold for a moment, then lower your hips back down. Repeat for a set number of repetitions, focusing on engaging your glutes and hamstrings.

5. Calf Raises: Stand behind the chair, holding onto the backrest for support. Rise up onto the

balls of your feet, lifting your heels off the ground. Hold for a moment at the top, then lower your heels back down. Repeat for a set number of repetitions, focusing on engaging your calf muscles.

Remember to maintain proper form and alignment throughout these exercises. Focus on engaging the targeted muscles and performing the movements with control. Adjust the intensity by increasing repetitions, adding weights, or slowing down the tempo. Incorporating these lower body sculpting and toning exercises into your Chair Pilates routine will help you achieve lean, strong, and well-defined lower body muscles.

- Abdominal And Waist Exercises

Strengthening and toning the abdominal muscles and waist area are essential for core stability, improved posture, and a defined midsection. Chair Pilates offers effective exercises that target these areas, helping you achieve a stronger core and a trimmer waistline. Here are some abdominal and waist exercises you can incorporate into your routine:

1. Seated Crunches: Sit tall on the chair with your feet flat on the floor and hands lightly resting behind your head, elbows wide. Inhale deeply, then as you exhale, engage your abdominal muscles and curl your chest towards your knees, performing a crunch. Inhale to release back to the starting position. Repeat for a set number of repetitions, focusing on controlled movements and avoiding strain on your neck.

2. Oblique Twists: Sit tall on the chair with your feet flat on the floor. Place your hands behind your head, elbows wide. Inhale deeply, then as you exhale, twist your torso to the right, bringing your right elbow towards your left knee. Inhale to release back to the starting position, then exhale and repeat on the other side. Continue alternating twists for a set number of repetitions, engaging your oblique muscles.

3. Side Bends: Sit on the edge of the chair with your feet flat on the floor and hands lightly resting on the sides of the chair seat. Inhale deeply, then as you exhale, slide your right hand down the side of the chair towards the floor, bending your torso to the right. Inhale to return to the upright position, then exhale and repeat on the other side. Continue alternating side bends for a set number of repetitions, feeling the stretch on your waistline.

4. Pelvic Tilts: Sit on the chair with your feet flat on the floor and hip-width apart. Place your hands on your hips. Inhale deeply, then as you exhale, tilt your pelvis forward, pressing your lower back into the chair. Hold for a few seconds, then inhale and release the tilt, allowing your lower back to arch slightly. Repeat the movement, focusing on engaging your abdominal muscles and maintaining control.

5. Waist Rotations: Sit tall on the chair with your feet flat on the floor and hands resting on your thighs. Inhale deeply, then as you exhale, rotate your torso to the right, keeping your hips stable.

Inhale to return to the center, then exhale and repeat the rotation to the left. Continue alternating waist rotations for a set number of repetitions, focusing on engaging your oblique muscles.

Remember to maintain proper alignment, breathe deeply throughout each exercise, and focus on engaging your abdominal muscles. Start with a comfortable range of motion and gradually increase the intensity as your core strength improves. By incorporating these abdominal and waist exercises into your Chair Pilates routine, you can sculpt and tone your midsection, leading to a stronger, more defined core.

- Back Strengthening and Posture Improvement

A strong and healthy back is crucial for maintaining proper posture, preventing back pain, and promoting overall spinal stability. Chair Pilates provides effective exercises to strengthen the muscles of your back and improve your posture. Here are some back strengthening and posture improvement exercises you can practice:

1. Seated Back Extension: Sit tall on the chair with your feet flat on the floor and hands resting lightly on the sides of the chair seat. Inhale deeply, then as you exhale, engage your back muscles and slowly arch your spine, lifting your chest and looking upwards. Inhale to release back to the starting position. Repeat for a set number of repetitions, focusing on the controlled movement of your spine.

2. Shoulder Blade Squeezes: Sit tall on the chair with your feet flat on the floor and hands resting lightly on the sides of the chair seat. Inhale deeply, then as you exhale, squeeze your shoulder blades together, retracting them towards your spine. Hold for a moment, then release. Repeat for a set number of repetitions, focusing on engaging your upper back muscles.

3. Seated Cat-Cow Stretch: Sit on the chair with your feet flat on the floor and hands resting on your thighs. Inhale deeply, then as you exhale, round your spine, tucking your chin towards

your chest and arching your back like a cat. Inhale to reverse the movement, lifting your chest and gently arching your back like a cow. Continue flowing between the cat and cow positions, focusing on the mobility and flexibility of your spine.

4. Upper Back Rotation: Sit tall on the chair with your feet flat on the floor and hands lightly resting on your shoulders, elbows wide. Inhale deeply, then as you exhale, rotate your upper body to the right, keeping your hips stable. Inhale to return to the center, then exhale and repeat the rotation to the left. Continue alternating upper back rotations for a set number of repetitions, focusing on engaging your back muscles and improving spinal mobility.

5. Back Stretch with Forward Fold: Sit tall on the chair with your feet flat on the floor. Inhale deeply, then as you exhale, hinge forward from your hips, allowing your upper body to fold forward. Relax your neck and let your arms dangle towards the floor. Hold this stretch for a few breaths, feeling the gentle stretch in your

back. Slowly roll back up to the starting position.

Remember to perform these exercises with control and focus on engaging the specific muscles of your back. Start with a comfortable range of motion and gradually increase the intensity as your back strength improves. By incorporating these back strengthening and posture improvement exercises into your Chair Pilates routine, you can develop a strong and stable back while promoting better posture and spinal alignment.

CHAPTER 3. CHAIR PILATES ROUTINES FOR DAILY PRACTICE

- Morning Energizer Routine

Starting your day with a Chair Pilates morning energizer routine is a fantastic way to awaken your body, boost your energy levels, and set a positive tone for the day ahead. This routine focuses on gentle movements and stretches that promote circulation, mobility, and overall vitality. Here's a sample morning energizer routine to help you kick-start your day:

1. Seated Cat-Cow Stretch: Sit tall on the chair with your feet flat on the floor and hands resting on your thighs. Inhale deeply, then as you exhale, round your spine, tucking your chin towards your chest and arching your back like a cat. Inhale to reverse the movement, lifting your chest and gently arching your back like a cow. Continue flowing between the cat and cow

positions, syncing your breath with each movement, and awakening your spine.

2. Shoulder Rolls: Sit tall on the chair with your feet flat on the floor. Inhale deeply, then as you exhale, roll your shoulders up towards your ears, back, and down in a smooth, circular motion. Repeat the shoulder rolls for a few rounds, then change direction. This movement helps release tension and improves shoulder mobility.

3. Chest Opener: Sit tall on the chair with your feet flat on the floor. Interlace your fingers behind your back, squeezing your shoulder blades together. Inhale deeply, then as you exhale, gently lift your interlaced hands away from your body, opening your chest. Feel the stretch across your chest and shoulders. Hold for a few breaths, then release.

4. Seated Twist: Sit tall on the chair with your feet flat on the floor. Inhale deeply, then as you exhale, twist your torso to the right, placing your left hand on the outside of your right thigh and your right hand on the backrest of the chair.

Inhale to lengthen your spine, and exhale to deepen the twist. Hold for a few breaths, then inhale to release and repeat on the other side. This movement stimulates digestion and awakens the spine.

5. Knee Lifts with Arm Reaches: Sit tall on the chair with your feet flat on the floor. Inhale deeply, then as you exhale, lift your right knee towards your chest while simultaneously reaching your left arm forward. Inhale to lower your leg and arm back down, then repeat on the other side. Continue alternating knee lifts and arm reaches for a few repetitions, feeling the engagement in your core and promoting coordination.

6. Seated Side Stretch: Sit tall on the chair with your feet flat on the floor. Inhale deeply, then as you exhale, raise your right arm overhead and lean gently to the left, feeling the stretch along your right side. Inhale to come back to the center, then exhale and repeat the stretch on the other side. Alternate side stretches for a few repetitions, promoting lateral mobility and awakening your entire body.

Remember to move with intention, focusing on deep, mindful breaths throughout the routine. Modify any movement as needed to suit your comfort and physical condition. The morning energizer routine should invigorate your body and prepare you for a productive and positive day ahead.

- *Midday Recharge Routine*

When the midday slump hits, a Chair Pilates recharge routine can help you refresh your mind and body, increase energy levels, and improve focus for the rest of the day. This routine focuses on rejuvenating movements and stretches to combat fatigue and promote mental clarity. Here's a sample midday recharge routine to revitalize your energy:

1. Seated Side Bend: Sit tall on the chair with your feet flat on the floor. Inhale deeply, then as you exhale, raise your right arm overhead and lean gently to the left, feeling the stretch along

your right side. Inhale to come back to the center, then exhale and repeat the stretch on the other side. Alternate side bends for a few repetitions, promoting lateral mobility and awakening your entire body.

2. Neck Stretches: Sit tall on the chair with your feet flat on the floor. Inhale deeply, then as you exhale, gently drop your chin towards your chest, feeling the stretch along the back of your neck. Hold for a few breaths, then slowly lift your head back to the upright position. Repeat this movement, then incorporate gentle side-to-side and ear-to-shoulder stretches to release tension in your neck and upper back.

3. Seated Forward Fold: Sit tall on the chair with your feet flat on the floor. Inhale deeply, then as you exhale, hinge forward from your hips, allowing your upper body to fold forward. Reach your hands towards your feet or the floor, relaxing your neck and shoulders. Hold this stretch for a few breaths, feeling the gentle stretch along the back of your legs and spine. Slowly roll back up to the starting position.

4. Deep Breathing: Sit tall on the chair with your feet flat on the floor. Place your hands on your abdomen. Inhale deeply through your nose, allowing your belly to expand and fill with air. Exhale slowly through your mouth, feeling your belly contract and empty. Continue this deep breathing pattern for a few minutes, focusing on calming your mind and releasing tension.

5. Seated Spinal Twist: Sit tall on the chair with your feet flat on the floor. Inhale deeply, then as you exhale, twist your torso to the right, placing your left hand on the outside of your right thigh and your right hand on the backrest of the chair. Inhale to lengthen your spine, and exhale to deepen the twist. Hold for a few breaths, then inhale to release and repeat on the other side. This movement stimulates digestion and awakens the spine.

6. Shoulder Rolls and Shakes: Sit tall on the chair with your feet flat on the floor. Inhale deeply, then as you exhale, roll your shoulders up towards your ears, back, and down in a smooth, circular motion. Repeat the shoulder rolls for a few rounds. Then, shake out your

arms and hands, allowing any tension to be released.

Remember to move with awareness, focusing on deep, mindful breaths throughout the routine. Modify any movement as needed to suit your comfort and physical condition. The midday recharge routine should invigorate your body, clear your mind, and help you regain focus and productivity for the remainder of the day.

- Evening Relaxation Routine

An evening relaxation routine using Chair Pilates is a wonderful way to unwind, release tension, and promote a peaceful transition from a busy day to a restful evening. This routine focuses on gentle movements, stretches, and breathing exercises that will help calm your mind, relax your body, and prepare you for a restorative night's sleep. Here's a sample evening relaxation routine to help you wind down:

1. Seated Deep Breathing: Sit tall on the chair with your feet flat on the floor. Place your hands on your abdomen. Inhale deeply through your nose, allowing your belly to expand and fill with air. Exhale slowly through your mouth, feeling your belly contract and empty. Continue this deep breathing pattern for a few minutes, focusing on relaxing your body and clearing your mind.

2. Neck and Shoulder Rolls: Sit tall on the chair with your feet flat on the floor. Inhale deeply, then as you exhale, gently drop your chin towards your chest, feeling the stretch along the back of your neck. Slowly begin to roll your head in a circular motion, bringing your right ear towards your right shoulder, then back, and continuing to the left side. Repeat this movement for a few rounds, allowing any tension in your neck and shoulders to release.

3. Seated Forward Fold: Sit tall on the chair with your feet flat on the floor. Inhale deeply, then as you exhale, hinge forward from your hips, allowing your upper body to fold forward.

Let your arms dangle towards the floor and relax your neck and shoulders. Breathe deeply and hold this stretch for a few breaths, allowing any tension in your back and legs to melt away. Slowly roll back up to the starting position.

4. Gentle Spine Twist: Sit tall on the chair with your feet flat on the floor. Inhale deeply, then as you exhale, twist your torso to the right, placing your left hand on the outside of your right thigh and your right hand on the backrest of the chair. Inhale to lengthen your spine, and exhale to deepen the twist. Hold for a few breaths, feeling the gentle release in your spine and lower back. Inhale to release and repeat the twist on the other side.

5. Seated Side Stretch: Sit tall on the chair with your feet flat on the floor. Inhale deeply, then as you exhale, raise your right arm overhead and lean gently to the left, feeling the stretch along your right side. Inhale to come back to the center, then exhale and repeat the stretch on the other side. Continue alternating side stretches for a few repetitions, promoting relaxation and a sense of release.

6. Seated Meditation: Sit tall on the chair with your feet flat on the floor. Close your eyes or soften your gaze. Bring your attention to your breath, allowing it to flow naturally. Focus on each inhale and exhale, letting go of any thoughts or worries that may arise. Stay in this state of meditation for a few minutes, enjoying the stillness and calmness it brings.

Remember to move gently and mindfully, honoring your body's limitations and avoiding any discomfort. This evening relaxation routine is designed to help you unwind and prepare for a peaceful evening and restorative sleep. As you finish the routine, carry the sense of relaxation and tranquility with you as you transition into your evening routine and bedtime.

Conclusion and Next Steps

Congratulations on completing your Chair Pilates journey! By incorporating the exercises, stretches, and routines outlined in this book, you have taken significant steps towards improving your strength, flexibility, balance, and overall well-being. As you conclude this book, it's important to reflect on your achievements and consider the next steps in your fitness journey.

Chair Pilates has provided you with a foundation of mindful movement and self-care. You have learned how to engage your core, strengthen your muscles, enhance flexibility, and improve your posture. These valuable skills can be applied not only during your Chair Pilates sessions but also in your everyday life.

Moving forward, consider the following next steps to maintain and expand upon your progress:

1. Consistency: Maintain a regular practice of Chair Pilates to continue reaping its benefits. Set aside dedicated time each week to engage in your exercises and routines. Consistency is key to progress and long-term results.

2. Progression: As you become more comfortable with the exercises, explore ways to challenge yourself further. Gradually increase the intensity, duration, or difficulty of your routines. Incorporate variations and new exercises to continually challenge and strengthen your body.

3. Listen to your Body: Pay attention to your body's cues and adjust your practice accordingly. Honor your limitations and modify exercises as needed. Remember that it's more important to move mindfully and with proper form rather than pushing yourself beyond your comfort zone.

4. Seek Guidance: If you desire further guidance or want to deepen your practice, consider working with a qualified Chair Pilates instructor. They can provide personalized

instruction, offer modifications for any specific needs or concerns, and help you progress safely.

5. Stay Active: Beyond Chair Pilates, maintain an active lifestyle that incorporates other forms of exercise and movement. Engage in activities you enjoy, such as walking, swimming, or cycling, to support your overall fitness and well-being.

Remember, Chair Pilates is not just a physical practice but also a journey of self-care and self-discovery. Be patient with yourself, celebrate your achievements, and embrace the process of continuous improvement. Enjoy the benefits of increased strength, flexibility, balance, and improved mind-body connection that Chair Pilates brings to your life.

Keep up the dedication, and may your Chair Pilates journey continue to bring you joy, vitality, and a sense of well-being.

9 798885 260 7232